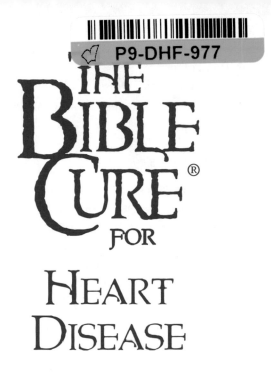

THE BIBLE CURE® FOR

HEART DISEASE

DON COLBERT, M.D.

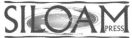

SILOAM PRESS

Living in Health—Body, Mind and Spirit

THE BIBLE CURE FOR HEART DISEASE
by Don Colbert, M.D.
Published by Siloam Press
A part of Strang Communications Company
600 Rinehart Road
Lake Mary, Florida 32746
www.siloampress.com

THE BIBLE CURE FOR HEART DISEASE
by Don Colbert, M.D.
Published by Siloam Press
A part of Strang Communications Company
600 Rinehart Road
Lake Mary, Florida 32746
www.siloampress.com

There's Hope for Your Heart

Hope beats the statistics and will help you overcome the threat of heart disease and attacks. In the United States, almost half a million people die annually due to heart attacks, and stroke is the No. 3 killer. Instead of becoming one of these statistics, you can take positive steps naturally and spiritually to beat heart disease. The risk of heart attacks and strokes can be greatly lessened through dietary and lifestyle changes.[1]

In fact, heart disease is one of the most treatable and preventable of all afflictions, despite the fact that it causes *almost half of all deaths* in the United States. That means you can fight back, overcome and win the battle. Through lifestyle changes, good nutrition, prayer and Scripture reading, you can respond in confident hope to this disease.

The initial symptoms and warning signs of heart disease are not a death sentence; they are a life warning. Change is required. Positive steps must be taken. The way you live and eat cannot remain the same if you want to have a healthy and strong heart. Take courage and be hopeful. You and God will prevail as you learn about the Bible Cure for heart disease.

This Bible Cure booklet will help you keep the temple of your body fit and healthy by preventing and overcoming heart disease. In these pages you will

*uncover God's divine plan of health
for body, soul and spirit
through modern medicine, good nutrition
and the medicinal power
of Scripture and prayer.*

Even if you're already suffering from heart disease, it's never too late to strengthen your faith in God and look to Him more fervently for the peace and healing you need. Throughout this booklet you'll find key Scriptures to help you focus on the healing power of God. These inspiring texts will guide your prayers and direct your thoughts toward God's plan of divine health for you in battling your heart disease or preventing it altogether. In this Bible Cure booklet, you will learn to overcome heart disease through the following chapters:

It is my prayer that these practical suggestions for health, nutrition and fitness will bring a new wholeness to your life. May they deepen your fellowship with God and strengthen your ability to worship and serve Him.

—DR. DON COLBERT

A BIBLE CURE PRAYER
FOR YOU

Heavenly Father, open my eyes to the natural and spiritual ways I can prevent and overcome heart disease. Give me the insight to apply all I learn with great wisdom. And grant me Your abiding peace, freeing me from all fear, anxiety and worry as I trust in Your sovereign will. In the name of the Healer, Jesus of Nazareth. Amen.

Chapter 1

Hope to Beat
the Statistics for Heart
Disease

H ave you ever considered the marvelous de-
sign and operation of your cardiovascular
system? It's the body's amazing superhighway. The
large arteries within it are much like interstate
roadways, and the smaller arteries are like small
streets and lanes. The primary function of the
whole system is to deliver oxygen and nutrients to
all the cells in your body and to remove cellular
debris and waste.

Each day your heart beats approximately
85,000 to 115,000 times. About 5,000 gallons of
blood travel 60,000 miles through blood vessels,
which include arteries, veins and capillaries. Thus
your heart will beat over two billion times if you
live an average lifespan, and it will pump over one

hundred billion gallons of blood. This superhighway system is truly wonderful.

Wouldn't it be a good idea to keep this blood superhighway free of traffic jams?

Building a Deadly Back-Up?

Yes, we might think of heart problems in terms of traffic flow—and a traffic jam. The worst contributor to a potentially deadly back-up is a condition called *arteriosclerosis,* which attacks the heart's blood vessels. The arteries that supply the heart with blood and nourishment are the coronary arteries. These are the most stressed arteries of the body because they're squeezed flat from the pumping action of the heart.

Arteriosclerosis is the hardening of these arteries due to excessive amounts of plaque. This plaque contains cholesterol, calcium and other fatty materials. You could compare plaque to rust in a pipe. As the plaque builds up in the arteries, blood flow is decreased to vital organs, including the heart and brain. This buildup can lead to an interruption of blood flow to an artery in the brain, causing a stroke. When blood flow is interrupted in a coronary artery, a heart attack occurs.

In general, heart disease also includes *congestive heart failure* (the heart is unable to pump out enough blood), *cardiomyopathy* (a disease of the heart muscle), *arrhythmia* (a disturbance of the heart rhythm) and *angina* (chest pains). Angina can occur when the coronary arteries are partially blocked. Such a blockage can even lead to a heart attack.

Freeing Up the Traffic

If arteriosclerosis is the cause of a deadly backup in the blood flow, you'll be happy to know that forces are at work in your body to free up the traffic. I can explain this best by breaking the process into two parts: 1) the problem of free radicals and 2) the way our bodies fight free radicals with antioxidants.

The problem: free radicals

A *free radical* isn't a terrorist trying to bomb our embassy; rather, it's a defective molecule that sends out molecular shrapnel, damaging the coronary artery cells and other cells in our bodies. To envision this problem, think about the oxidation process. Burn wood in a fireplace and smoke is a by-product. Likewise, when you metabolize food into energy, oxygen oxidizes (or burns) the food in order to produce energy. This process does not create smoke like burning wood in a fireplace, but it does produce dangerous by-products known as free radicals. These are molecules that have set electrons roaming free to do damage in other cells.

These erratic electrons can damage cells' DNA, and in some cases can cause cells to mutate, forming cancerous growths. With regard to heart disease, the problem is that free radicals wreak havoc on artery linings. You see, the lining of the coronary arteries is comprised of very sensitive cells that can easily sustain damage by free radicals produced from cigarette smoke, hypertension, excessive stress, high cholesterol, high lipoprotein-a and others.

Don't you realize that all of you together are the temple of God and that the Spirit of God lives in you? God will bring ruin upon anyone who ruins this temple. For God's temple is holy, and you Christians are that temple.
—1 CORINTHIANS 3:16–17

So, free radicals are the enemies of our heart and of our bodies' cells in general. Some estimates calculate that the cells in our bodies sustain over 10,000 hits from free radicals each day.

The solution: antioxidants

God's Bible cure in winning the battle against heart disease includes a powerful weapon against free radicals—*antioxidants*. They're amazing substances that prevent oxidation and block or repair free-radical reactions in our bodies.

The heart is the hardest-working organ in the body. Since the coronary arteries sustain more wear and tear than other arteries, they also need to be constantly repaired. Antioxidants are extremely important in preventing heart disease due to their blocking and repairing functions. Powerful antioxidants called *proanthocyanidins* abound in pine bark extract (which is pycnogenol) and grape seed extract.

Millions of small cracks and damaged areas occur inside the artery walls. When the body does not have adequate amounts of antioxidants, especially vitamin C and E, in order to repair the lining of damaged blood vessels, it will use cholesterol and lipoproteins to repair the lining instead. This forms fatty streaks on the blood vessels and leads to the hard places lined with plaque.

However, adequate amounts of vitamin C and vitamin E, pycnogenol and grape seed extract can prevent these cracks from occurring in the first place.

Picture it this way: Imagine repairing a house after a tornado has damaged the roof and knocked down walls. If you didn't have the money to repair the roof and walls properly, and you merely patched them with the inexpensive materials at hand, the next storm might well destroy your dwelling for good.

Likewise, if you have inadequate antioxidants in your diet and you are damaging your blood vessels with smoking, stress or a fatty diet, your body will then repair the lining of your blood vessels with a cholesterol patch instead of using proper materials. Consequently, more plaque is formed. If this continues over decades, the cholesterol plaque builds up in your blood vessels, creating arteriosclerosis, which can lead to a heart attack. This certainly isn't God's will for you!

> Dear friend, I am praying that all is well with you and that your body is as healthy as I know your soul is.
>
> —3 JOHN 2

6

For a healthy heart, don't forget your vitamin C. It's a very important antioxidant for repairing damage to the coronary arteries. It helps to increase the production of collagen and elastin, both of which add stability to our blood vessels. Collagen produced without vitamin C is weaker and causes blood vessels to become fragile. Scurvy results from an extremely depleted supply of vitamin C reserves in the body. This condition causes a gradual breakdown of collagen, leading to a breakdown in blood vessels, resulting in hemorrhaging.

✓ A BIBLE CURE HEALTHFACT

While many animals can create their own vitamin C, people cannot. We must replenish it daily through our diet. Unfortunately, much of our food is so processed that very little vitamin C remains on our plate. Corn is a major source of vitamin C, but many people are allergic to it. While most of us may have enough vitamin C to prevent scurvy, we don't have enough to win the war against arteriosclerosis.

HEALTHFACT HEALTHFACT HEALTHFACT HEALTHFACT HEALTHFACT HEALTHFACT HEALTHFACT

We will talk more about the benefits of vitamin C in the next chapter.

Living With Faith and Hope

According to American Heart Association statistics (1996), one in two deaths in the United States is related to heart disease. However, the encouraging news is that of the twelve million Americans who have suffered from angina (chest pain), heart attack and other forms of coronary disease, the majority are still living. And from 1986 to 1996 the death rate from coronary heart disease declined 27 percent.[1]

While these statistics are encouraging, we can also be optimistic because heart disease is one of the most preventable of all degenerative diseases. Furthermore, we can take great hope in the reality that God is our Healer (Exod. 15:26). Nutrition and lifestyle changes are the cornerstones in keeping it at bay. Prayer is a great resource in building our hope and opening our lives up to God's healing power.

The major contributors to heart disease are unhealthy diet, lack of exercise and obesity. Clearly, these three factors are within our control. And you can make a decision to put your faith and trust in God's Spirit to help you implement the steps you need to take to eat healthy, exercise and lose weight if you are overweight.

Yes, there is hope for this amazing, hardworking superhighway system in your body. It can keep the nutrients flowing for years and years with no breakdowns. So I encourage you to live each day in faith and hope, while taking some important preventive steps right away. Make this your hope:

> I wait quietly before God, for my hope is in him. He alone is my rock and my salvation, my fortress where I will not be shaken.
>
> —PSALM 62:5–6

In the chapters to come, you'll learn what you can do to defeat our No. 1 killer.

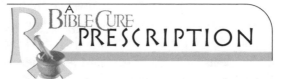

What Do You Think?

Rank from most important (1) to least important (5) the factors that give you hope:

__ God is my strength, healer and rock of my hope.

__ Good nutrition can reduce the risk of heart attack.

__ Faith and prayer build hope in the God who guides me through making healthy decisions about diet and nutrition.

__ Statistics are showing that heart disease is one of the most preventable of all diseases.

__ The actual number of deaths attributed to heart disease is declining.

Chapter 2

Hope to Overcome
the Risk of Heart Disease

You have some important choices to make. You can put yourself at greater risk for a heart attack or you can take steps now to reduce your risk. God has put some powerful resources and information in your hands for living a healthier life. But you must decide to use what you know and implement positive steps both in the natural and spiritual realms to prevent heart disease.

✓ A BIBLE CURE HEALTHFACT

A simple warning sign of heart disease is a diagonal crease in the ear lobes. If one does have creases in the ear lobes, there is a strong probability of significant arteriosclerosis in the coronary arteries.[1]

HEALTHFACT HEALTHFACT HEALTHFACT HEALTHFACT HEALTHFACT HEALTHFACT HEALTHFACT

In this chapter, you will learn about the factors that put you at risk and what to do about them. Make a decision now to implement what you learn.

A Bit Concerned?

One significant factor affecting your risk for heart disease is being overweight. Are you concerned about your weight? Your weight may be partially dictated by heredity. It may be a hereditary condition over which you have little control.

But here's the good news: my experience in medicine tells me that no matter what condition your heart is in today, there is hope for health and recovery in the future. Yes, even if your parents or grandparents suffered from heart disease. If you'll simply follow the list of recommendations in this chapter, you will discover that clogged arteries and a weak heart can often be reversed without surgery. And remember God's Word with regard to everything I'm saying. Health and healing are what the Lord has in mind for you, just as He told the prophet long ago:

> I will give you back your health and heal
> your wounds, says the LORD.
> —JEREMIAH 30:17

Of course, if you are indeed serious about reversing or preventing heart disease, you'll have to change the way you eat, exercise and even think. But don't try to change your lifestyle completely all at once. Just take some new steps, day by day, to a healthier heart.

A BIBLE CURE PRAYER
FOR YOU

Almighty God, just as You can give me a new heart spiritually, help me to strengthen and care for my natural heart by taking healthy, preventive steps through diet, nutrition, supplements and exercise. Through Your Spirit, help me to be wise in implementing the knowledge that You have provided through Your grace. Amen.

First, Another Lesson on Antioxidants

In the previous chapter I told you about the problem caused by free radicals roaming through your body. I mentioned that antioxidants are the solution, but I'm sure you'd like a little more detail, wouldn't you? So first let me stress that in order to minimize the amount of damage to the lining of your coronary blood vessels (the *endothelium*), you should take adequate amounts of antioxidants, especially these:

- Vitamin C (1,000–3,000 mg. daily)
- Vitamin E (400–800 I.U. daily)
- Grape seed extract (50–200 mg. daily)
- Pine bark extract (50–200 mg. daily)
- Beta carotene (25,000 I.U. daily)
- Selenium (200 mcg. daily)

By adding adequate amounts of Vitamin C to your diet you will increase the production of collagen and elastin, which make your arteries stronger. Vitamin C is responsible for regenerating oxidized vitamin E in the body. Simply put, vitamin E is much more effective in our bodies when vitamin C is present. Vitamin E improves your circulation, normal blood clotting, reduces blood pressure and strengthens the walls of your capillaries.

Vitamin C helps keep cholesterol from being oxidized, too, a function that is directly related to preventing arteriosclerosis. You see, oxidized cholesterol comes from processed foods, animal products (such as red meat and scrambled eggs) and environmental chemicals (such as pesticides, DDT, chlorine and fluoride). Stress can also cause regular cholesterol to be converted to oxidized cholesterol.

When you eat the right things and stop eating the wrong things, you are contributing to your health in more ways than one. You are also strengthening the life of the Spirit within you, through your honoring of the one who "owns" you.

> *And God said, "Look! I have given you the seed-bearing plants throughout the earth and all the fruit trees for your food. And I have given all the grasses and other green plants to the animals and birds for their food." And so it was.*
> —Genesis 1:29–30

Don't you know that your body is the temple of the Holy Spirit, who lives in you and was given to you by God? You do not belong to yourself, for God bought you with a price. So you must honor God with your body.
—1 Corinthians 6:19–20

15

More Things You Can Do

Now I'll just list some of the other things you can do to help lower your risk for heart disease. Think of them as five steps to a longer life.

Limit your fat consumption. Take a dramatic step here as soon as possible! Especially reduce your intake of the saturated fats found in red meat, pork (especially bacon), whole milk, cheese, butter, ice cream, fried foods and chicken skins. Even more dangerous to the health of your heart than saturated fats are hydrogenated fats, found in margarine, peanut butter, processed foods, pastries, cookies and donuts—they can even be found in many so-called "health products." I recommend limiting the amount of fat consumed to less than 30 percent of daily calories.

Did you know that eating fat is forbidden in the Bible? God commands: "You must never eat any fat or blood. This is a permanent law for you and all your descendants, wherever they may live" (Lev. 3:17).

God created our bodies, and He knows how they have been designed to function best. This verse likely refers to the harmful fats called *low-density lipoproteins (LDL)*. The good fats you should consume are the *omega-3 fatty acids,* which include flaxseed oil and cold saltwater fish, such as salmon, tuna, halibut, cod and mackerel. In general, the more omega-3 oils that individuals eat, the less coronary artery disease they experience.

Substituting extra-virgin olive oil and canola oil for butter and cream decreases your risk of developing arteriosclerosis. This is no doubt the reason why the Mediterranean Diet, or a diet high in olive oils, is associated with lower risk of heart disease. Here's how this type of diet typically looks:

The Mediterranean Diet

Most of the following ingredients, which are a part of the Mediterranean diet, are consumed daily.

- *Olive oil.* Replaces most fats, oils, butter, and margarine. It is used in salads as well as for cooking. Extra-virgin olive oil raises levels of the good cholesterol *(HDL)* and may strengthen the immune system.
- *Breads.* Consumed daily and prepared as dark, chewy, crusty loaves. Eat whole grain breads and avoid white processed bread.

- *Pasta, rice, couscous, bulgar, potatoes.* Often served with fresh vegetables and herbs sautéed in olive oil. Occasionally served with small quantities of lean beef. Dark rice preferred.
- *Grains.* Consumed regularly, such as wheat bran (one-half cup, four to five times weekly); alternate with a cereal such as Bran Buds (one-half cup) or other cereals that contain oat bran (one-third cup).
- *Fruits.* Preferably raw, two to three pieces daily; and nuts, especially walnuts and almonds, at least 10 per day.
- *Beans.* Include pintos, great northern, navy and kidney beans. Beans and lentil soups are very popular (prepared with a small amount of olive oil). Have at least one-half cup of beans, three to four times weekly.
- *Vegetables.* Dark green variety, especially in salads. Eat at least one serving of the following daily: cabbage, broccoli, cauliflower, turnip greens, mustard greens, carrots, spinach or sweet potatoes.
- *Cheese and yogurt.* Cheese may be grated on soups or a small wedge may be com-

bined with a piece of fruit for dessert. Use the reduced-fat varieties. (The fat-free cheeses often taste like rubber.) The best yogurt is fat-free, but not frozen.

Include the following foods in your diet only a few times weekly:

- *Fish.* The healthiest fish are cold-water varieties such as cod, salmon, and mackerel. These are high in omega-3 fatty acids.
- *Poultry.* Eaten two to three times weekly. Eat white breast meat with the skin removed.
- *Eggs.* Eaten only in small amounts (two to three per week).
- *Red meat.* Only rarely, on an average of three times a month. Use only lean cuts with the fat trimmed. Use in small amounts as an additive to spice up soup or pasta. (Note: the severe restriction of red meat in the Mediterranean diet is a radical departure from the American diet, but it is a major contributor to the low rates of cancer and heart disease found in these countries.)

Let Go of Type A Behavior

Are you the Type A type? You are, if you're often impatient, extremely competitive and pretty aggressive in most everything you do. Type A's have twice the risk of heart disease as compared with non-Type A folks. We know that constant, excessive anger, worry, stress and anxiety pump up the adrenalin levels, raise the blood pressure and thereby exert heavier loads on the heart and circulatory system. The risk of heart disease—especially heart attack—increases for the Type A types.

Comedian Lily Tomlin put it nicely: "The trouble with the rat race is that even if you win, you're still a rat." Many of us are so caught up in the race to get ahead that we leave our health behind. Our hearts suffer under the stress and tension of trying to be on top and at the head of every line.

Words satisfy the soul as food satisfies the stomach; the right words on a person's lips bring satisfaction. Those who love to talk will experience the consequences, for the tongue can kill or nourish life.
—PROVERBS 18:20–21

Test yourself for Type A behaviors by the descriptions below that describe you accurately.

❑ I feel stressed and pressured to get things done.

❑ Relaxing is hard for me.

❑ It bothers me when I don't get a task completed in the amount of time I have allotted.

❑ When others do their jobs right, my life is easier.

❑ I have trouble sitting at a long stoplight.

❑ People who don't know what they want stress me.

❑ Hobbies like fishing or bowling aren't active enough for me.

❑ Acquiring assets and being financially secure are important to me.

❑ I put off family activities for important meetings.

❑ I want to be adequate and capable in all possible respects.

The more items checked, the more entrenched you are as a Type A personality. Type A personalities usually feel urgent about what they are doing, become angry when frustrated, and express aggressive, hostile or competitive behavior. They are generally dissatisfied with their own performance and the performance of others. Type A personalities need to relax, work on their communication skills, have fun and enjoy what God has created including other people.

Type A personalities are always in a hurry and try to accomplish too many activities or tasks in a fixed amount of time. They tend to accelerate daily activities

> *You must never eat any fat or blood. This is a permanent law for you and all your descendants, wherever they may live.*
> —LEVITICUS 3:17

(speeding up speech and finishing the sentences of others in a conversation; walking and eating quickly; doing two or three tasks at the same time) and often engage in two or more conversations at the same time. Unfortunately, they also develop a drive toward self-destruction (usually unconscious). Yet this drive seems to help them relieve their stress, since they look forward to finally escaping life's treadmill.[2]

The Bible Cure offers some important counsel for Type A personalities. For example, consider Jesus' wise prescription for lowering stress found in Matthew 6:19–34. Why not read through that passage now, focusing specifically on verses 32–34?

> Your heavenly Father already knows all your needs, and he will give you all you need from day to day if you live for him and make the Kingdom of God your primary concern. So don't worry about tomorrow, for tomorrow will bring its own worries. Today's trouble is enough for today.

Don't Smoke!

The most important lifestyle modification in preventing arteriosclerosis, if you're a smoker, is to stop smoking! But even nonsmokers need to avoid second-hand smoke. Cigarette smoke fills the air with over four thousand chemicals, fifty of which are cancer causing. These chemicals trigger significant free radical reactions, which damage the linings of the arteries or damage healthy cholesterol and form oxidized cholesterol.

Smoking also causes blood platelets to clump together and so raises fibrinogen levels, which increases your risk of both heart attack and stroke.

Reduce Your Stress

Who would dispute that our emotions affect our physical bodies? When we're overly stressed, destructive changes occur in the chemical makeup of our brains and circulatory systems. So reducing stress does more than make you more emotionally healthy. It makes you more physically healthy as well.

Exercise Regularly

The average heart rate of an unconditioned heart at rest is about seventy-five to eighty-five beats per minute. A well-conditioned heart beats approximately sixty beats per minute. Since the unconditioned heart beats approximately twenty beats more per minute, that is an extra twelve hundred beats per hour, almost twenty-nine thousand extra beats per day, and over ten million extra beats per year!

Naturally, it would great if your heart could do a little less work during your lifetime. The way to lower your heart rate is to exercise regularly, for at least thirty minutes, four times per week.

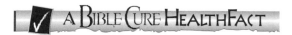

A [person] awaiting death is not disturbed by many stress factors that upset people. He is not upset because his neighbor's chickens are scratching up his flower bed; his arthritis is not worsened because the taxes on his house have been raised; his blood pressure is not raised because his employer discharged him; he doesn't get a migraine headache because his wife burned his toast; and his ulcerative colitis doesn't flare up because the stock market goes down ten points. The crucified soul is not frustrated. The man who willingly, cheerfully and daily presents himself as a living sacrifice can excellently adapt to the severest situations and, with Paul, be more than conqueror.[3]

Finally, a Better Way to Live

In 1 Corinthians 15:31, the apostle Paul said, "I die daily" (NKJV). In effect, Paul was living what

25

might be called the crucified life. It's a way of approaching each day in peace, knowing that our lives and futures are in God's hands, knowing that we have let Him have our egos and everything else that ought to matter so much less to us than God's kingdom. I highly recommend this way of living. It's good for the heart and it's good for the soul.

The most wonderful thing about the crucified life is that we can make it ours at any moment.

We simply choose to adjust our focus. In the face of potential stress, imminent worry or intruding anxiety, we can remind ourselves, I am crucified with Christ. Then we rest in His love.

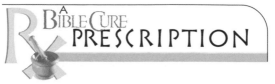

A BIBLE CURE PRESCRIPTION

Healthy First Steps

You can find hope for a healthy heart today by taking these simple first steps. Check off the ones you are now taking, and underline the ones you need to start immediately.

❑ Take vitamin C and vitamin E.

❑ Limit fat.

❑ Follow the Mediterranean Diet.

❑ Reduce stress.

❑ Don't smoke.

❑ Stop worrying so much.

❑ Exercise regularly.

❑ Consult with your physician or nutritional doctor.

❑ Pray for God's guidance and healing.

Chapter 3

Hope for Lower Cholesterol

Y ou sit on the cold metal chair watching your doctor look over the results of your blood test. He's frowning, and you're getting more and more nervous. Finally, he speaks: "Your LDL level is well over 250, and I'm afraid your lipoprotein-a levels are at 40. Looks to me like you're at risk for a heart attack unless you do something about your cholesterol."

You lean back in the chair, your head spinning. *So what do I do now?* Your first step is to pray, asking God for His healing power to touch you physically and wisdom to guide your steps. God has not only promised to heal (Exod. 15:26), He has also promised to be with you through every circumstance in life (Ps. 23; Heb. 13:5). God is your strength and your shield. Remember His promise: "For God has said, 'I will never fail you. I will never forsake you.'" That is why we can say with confidence, "The Lord is my helper, so I will not be afraid. What can mere mortals do to me?" (Heb. 13:5–6).

Battling Killer Cholesterol

Actually, your natural and spiritual diagnosis is hopeful. You have a great deal of control over the cholesterol flowing through your arteries, and, therefore, you have great power to promote and maintain healthy arteries and a healthy heart. Even if you have heart disease, clogged arteries can be reversed without surgery. And God is at work in you to strengthen your hope and heal your body.

> *If you will listen carefully to the voice of the LORD your God and do what is right in his sight, obeying his commands and laws, then I will not make you suffer the diseases I sent on the Egyptians; for I am the LORD who heals you.*
> —EXODUS 15:26

Begin by realizing that the health of your heart depends upon the health of your arteries. Yes, cholesterol is the enemy—but not all cholesterol is bad. Two different types are battling over your arteries: HDL (high-density lipoprotein), which is the good form, and LDL (low-density lipoprotein), which is the bad form. LDL cholesterol is the plaque-producing enemy that, if permitted, can eventually cause a heart attack. But you have a heroic warrior launching attacks against this killer. HDL battles the bad cholesterol in a tireless quest to keep your arteries plaque-free and healthy.

Now, what about that lipoprotein your doctor mentioned? Cholesterol is carried in the blood by this form of protein. There are many different kinds of lipoproteins, including HDL and LDL, but the worst is *lipoprotein-a*. High levels of it are associated with ten times the risk of heart disease. This is because lipoprotein-a has an uncanny ability to stick to the walls of the arteries. If your levels of lipoprotein-a are measured below twenty, then your risk of heart disease is low. However, levels above forty are associated with a dangerously high risk of heart disease.

High cholesterol is usually due to dietary or lifestyle factors, but it may also be due to genetic conditions such as *familial hypercholesterolemia* (an excessive amount of cholesterol in the blood). Dietary guidelines are the most important prescription for lowering cholesterol levels. In order to avoid or reduce high cholesterol, you should eat less saturated fat and cholesterol, and reduce your intake of animal products overall. You should also decrease the amount of processed foods and avoid sugar. High-fiber foods, including whole grains, fruits, vegetables and legumes, are helpful in lowering cholesterol. Maintaining your ideal body weight is also very important in lowering your serum cholesterol level.

Let's get more specific regarding the things you can do about your cholesterol levels. Be certain to consult with your physician before taking these steps. We'll look at them as a two-step process.

Step #1: Doing it with diet

This first step is easy and economical. It doesn't require high medical bills and won't cost you a trip to the operating room. Just look at your diet and make an effort to decrease or avoid fried foods, red meats, hot dogs and other cured meats. Also reduce the intake of eggs, high fat dairy products, butter, cream, lard and other saturated fats.

31

Finally, cut back and then eliminate high-sugar foods, including ice cream, pies, cakes, cookies, candies, white bread, processed foods, refined cereals, chips and other chip-like snack foods, salty foods and soft drinks.[1]

There are all kinds of wonderful things to add to your diet in the process! Eat primarily fruits, vegetables and whole grains. Also enjoy lean meats such as chicken breast, turkey breast and fish (but remember to peel the skins off the chicken and turkey). Using extra-virgin olive oil or canola oil instead of other vegetable oils also benefits your health.

> *You must serve only the LORD your God. If you do, I will bless you with food and water, and I will keep you healthy.*
> —EXODUS 23:25

A high-fiber diet can really help you beat heart disease. That's because fiber helps bind the bad cholesterol so it is excreted through the colon. I personally use fresh flax seeds ground in a coffee grinder—five teaspoons, two to three times a day. These can be taken with meals sprinkled on your food, or you may use psyllium husk, oat bran or modified citrus pectin.

I also place all my patients with high cholesterol on flaxseed oil, one tablespoon, one to two times a day.

And don't forget the omega-3 fatty acids, such as fish oil. They lower the levels of *triglycerides* and the LDL cholesterol. Also, canola and olive oil contain oleic acid, which is a form of fatty acid much less prone to being damaged by free radicals. This is probably the reason why people who eat the Mediterranean Diet, which has high amounts of olive oil, have significantly less heart disease. I recommend three (500 mg.) gel capsules of fish oil three times daily with meals. Fish oil capsules should contain combined omega-3 fatty acids EPH and DHA. You may need to take pancreatic enzymes to digest the fish oil properly.

Finally, be sure your diet contains enough magnesium and potassium. These two minerals are extremely important in the healthy functioning of the cardiovascular system. Many people in the U.S. are deficient in magnesium because they eat too many processed foods and not enough fruits and vegetables.

Magnesium is found primarily in seeds, nuts, whole grains and green leafy vegetables. But these are foods the average American rarely eats. Magnesium dilates the coronary arteries, improving blood flow and oxygen to the heart. Magnesium also helps to prevent arrhythmia. The best forms include magnesium glycinate, taurate or aspartate. The recommended daily allowance for magnesium is 350 milligrams for men and 280 for women. However, pregnant women should get 320 milligrams in their diets.

Magnesium must be balanced with potassium so that heart muscle contractions will be regulated properly. Researchers at a heart institute in Israel found that potassium levels were severely low among patients with heart arrhythmias, which caused medical experts to conclude that potassium is an important mineral for a healthy functioning heart.[2]

It's best get the potassium you need from dietary sources such as lean meats, raw vegetables, fruits (especially citrus fruits, bananas and avocados), potatoes and dandelion greens. Do not take potassium supplements without consulting your doctor first.

How Much Resistance?

When people are confronted with the need to make significant changes—especially in their eating habits—they often experience quite a bit of inward resistance. As the apostle Paul said: "I don't understand myself at all, for I really want to do what is right, but I don't do it. Instead, I do the very thing I hate" (Rom. 7:15). Through God's Spirit we will have the strength to make changes and stick with them. Fortunately, Paul didn't finish his thought there. He went on to say: "Who will free me from this life that is dominated by sin? Thank God! The answer is in Jesus Christ our Lord" (Rom. 7:24–25).

God understood exactly what we would face in this life. He knew well that weaknesses of will power, physical strength and emotional stamina

> *For God has not given us a spirit of fear and timidity, but of power, love, and self-discipline.*
> —2 TIMOTHY 1:7

would challenge us continually. So He provided the complete answer for us through Jesus Christ. If you try to do it alone, you may well fail. But if you ask for God's help, He will never fail you! He will strengthen your desire to do right and your determination to get it done. Then He will give you the power to make it happen. Jesus Christ is ALL you need!

Write a list of all the weaknesses you need God to help you overcome, and date each item.

1. _____

2. _____

3. _____

4. _____

5. _____

Now, go back through this list, and thank God ahead of time for His help. When your prayer for help is answered, draw a line through the need and record the date you received your answer. You may be delightfully surprised to see how faithful God really is. This will prove a wonderful record of the goodness of God in your life.

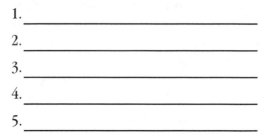

Step #2: Trying nutritional therapy

If this diet does the trick, you won't need this step. However, if your diet isn't effectively reducing your cholesterol, you may wish to begin nutritional therapy. Check with your doctor, but here are some of my general recommendations:

- *Vitamin B / Niacin.* Niacin is a B vitamin (B_3) that lowers the bad LDL cholesterol and raises the good HDL cholesterol. In the form of inositol hexaniacinate, niacin lowers LDL cholesterol, lipoprotein-a and triglycerides. None of the available cholesterol-lowering medicines are able to lower lipoprotein-a, but the B vitamin niacin can lower lipoprotein-a levels up to 36 percent! Start with 500 milligrams of inositol hexaniacinate, three times a day and work up to 1000 milligrams, three times a day.

Very important warning: You should not use niacin, however, if you have liver disease or elevated liver enzymes. If you take niacin or inositol hexaniacinate, have your liver functions monitored by a physician every three months. Do not take niacin with other cholesterol-lowering drugs, such as Mevacor, Lipitor, Zocor and Pravachol. Also, niacin must be used with caution in diabetics since it can impair blood sugar control.

Pantethine is a form of B_5, and it is involved in the transportation of fats to and from cells. Pantethine is able to lower cholesterol, triglycerides and LDL cholesterol. HDL is increased while taking pantethine. Pantethine actually inhibits the manufacture of cholesterol and allows fats to be used as energy. Diabetics can be treated with pantethine because it does not interfere with insulin.

- *Vitamin C.* This vitamin may increase HDL levels and may help to lower lipoprotein-a. It should be taken in a dose of approximately 1000 milligrams, three times a day. I prefer the buffered form of vitamin C. Unfortunately, many people are allergic to vitamin C and need to be desensitized using N.A.E.T. (Nambudripad's Allergy Elimination Techniques). This therapy is used by physicians trained in this specialized technique. It is natural, drugless, painless and a non-invasive method of eliminating allergies one at a time.[3]
- *Vitamin E.* This vitamin is extremely important in preventing arteriosclerosis since it prevents free radical damage to the blood vessels. Low levels of vitamin E in the blood are more predictive of a heart attack than high blood cholesterol or high blood pressure. The recommended daily

allowance for vitamin E is 12 International Units for women (8 mg.), and 15 International Units for men (10 mg.).

Two studies show how well vitamin E reduces heart disease. The first looked at over 87,000 nurses. It showed that the nurses who took 100 International Units of vitamin E daily for over two years had a 41 percent lower risk of heart disease than nurses who did not use vitamin E.[4] Another study looked at 156 men who had had coronary bypass graft surgery. The subjects who had taken over 100 International Units of vitamin E developed less coronary artery disease than those who took less than 100 International Units of vitamin E.[5]

- *Garlic preparations.* These are able to lower serum cholesterol levels as well as LDL levels. HDL levels are raised, but triglycerides are lowered. Garlic should be taken in a dose of 400 milligrams three times a day, or an equivalent of 4,000 micrograms of allicin potential A, taken three times a day.
- *Gugulipid.* This is an extract from the mukulmyrrh tree from India. Gugulipid

is able to lower both LDL cholesterol and triglycerides and raise HDL cholesterol levels. The standard dose of gugulipid is 500 milligrams, three times a day.

Keeping the Blessing

Anyone who loses his good health will tell you that it is a precious gift from God. Too many of us are guilty of squandering this treasure by not caring for our bodies as we should. When it's gone, we live with regrets. How much better to make healthy lifestyle choices before we lose our good health?

"Look to your health; and if you have it, praise God, and value it next to a good conscience." These were the words of an English writer, Izaak Walton. He also said that health is a blessing from God that money cannot buy. It's true. All the money in the world cannot replace your good health once you have lost it. Be grateful for the gift of good health that you have, and renew your commitment to keep it. It is a precious treasure!

> That good thing that was committed to you, keep by the Holy Spirit who dwells in us.
>
> —2 TIMOTHY 1:14, NKJV

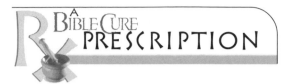

Winning the War
Against High Cholesterol

Circle when you will take these steps:

Decrease my consumption of processed foods and increase my consumption of high-fiber foods.

Now   Later   Never

Eliminate fatty foods and fried foods from my diet, replacing them with fruits and vegetables.

Now   Later   Never

Increase my use of vitamins C and E.

Now   Later   Never

Eat garlic or take garlic supplements.

Now   Later   Never

Use other supplements, such as gugulipid and pantethine.

Now   Later   Never

If you circled NOW for each item above, take hope. You are starting to win the war against heart disease.

Chapter 4

Hope for
Ending Angina

Y ou do not have to live with the pain of angina. God has provided both natural and spiritual ways for you to end your angina. In this chapter we will explore many natural ways that God has created for overcoming pain from angina, and we will build hope with the spiritual ways that God provides for our healing.

The prayer of the psalmist can become yours today: " I am suffering and in pain. Rescue me, O God, by your saving power. Then I will praise God's name with singing, and I will honor him with thanksgiving" (Ps. 69:29–30). God understands your pain and wills to deliver and heal you. Claim this Bible cure promise: "The Lord nurses them when they are sick and eases their pain and discomfort" (Ps. 41:3). Seek God's healing through this prayer:

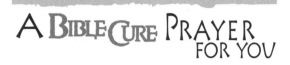

A BIBLE CURE PRAYER FOR YOU

Almighty God, remove the pain of angina from my heart. Give me wisdom as I take steps in the natural to end this pain. Touch my heart muscle with Your healing power and nurse me through this sickness, pain and discomfort. Heal me, O God, for Your glory and name's sake (Jer. 15:18). Amen.

Is the Pain Getting You Down?

Some people think that faith in God comes from great emotion—that it's something that only a few people have. They are mistaken. Faith is a choice to believe God's Word despite everything else to the contrary—even your pain. That doesn't mean that you pretend your pain isn't there. Instead, you choose to believe in God's power to heal.

One of the more grievous forms of heart disease is angina, a condition that causes spasmodic, suffocating pain in the chest. It produces significant discomfort and often stirs up a good deal of anxiety in those who suffer with it on a daily basis. Exertion triggers the pressure-like chest pain of angina. It's due to a lack of oxygen to the heart muscle. Many times angina is the first sign of an impending heart attack.

One of the foundational problems involved with angina and other heart-disease conditions is poor circulation due to arteriosclerosis, which inhibits the flow of blood and thus oxygen in our bodies. We will discuss this later in this chapter.

> *Praise the LORD, I tell myself; with my whole heart, I will praise his holy name. Praise the LORD, I tell myself, and never forget the good things he does for me. He forgives all my sins and heals all my diseases.*
> —PSALM 103:1–3

What is the cause of this oxygen deficit? The heart uses fat as its primary source of fuel. But when too much fat is sent to the heart, fatty acid will begin to accumulate within the coronary arteries. The heart doesn't receive adequate blood flow due to plaque buildup, and this, along with the lack of oxygen, brings on the pain.

Thankfully, you can take positive steps to win the battle against this painful condition. The following nutrients help convert fatty acids into energy. Consult with your physician and discuss with your doctor how these nutrients can help.

Carnitine. This nutrient helps transport fatty acids within the cells so they can be broken down into energy. This prevents toxic fatty acid metabolites from being produced. A decrease of carnitine will cause a decrease in energy production. L-carnitine should be supplemented in a dose of 500 milligrams, three times a day.

Coenzyme Q_{10}. This antioxidant is very important in energy production. It helps decrease the frequency of angina attacks because it causes an increase in the force of the contractions of the heart. It should be taken in a dose of approximately 100 milligrams, two to three times a day.

Hawthorn. Here's an herb that improves blood flow to the heart, as well as oxygen to the heart, by dilating the coronary arteries. It is very effective in the treatment of heart failure and arrhythmia. I recommend taking a capsule of 100 to 300 milligrams of herbal extract capsules, three times a day.

Khella. This is another herb that has been used for thousands of years in the treatment of heart disease. It helps to dilate the coronary arteries and thus relieve angina. Take it in a dose of 100 milligrams, three times a day.

Magnesium. This mineral is extremely important in preventing angina that is caused by spasms of the coronary artery. Magnesium can be taken at a dose of 400 milligrams, three times a day. (Note: If taking magnesium causes you to develop diarrhea, decrease your dosage, or start with 400 milligrams of magnesium a day and gradually increase the dose to 400 milligrams three times a day.)

One more word about magnesium. If you're suffering with congestive heart failure or arrhythmia, magnesium should help you. In fact, magnesium deficiency is very common in those who have congestive heart failure. Certain conventional drugs for treating congestive heart failure, such as Lanoxin and various diuretics, can deplete magnesium levels.

All individuals who have experienced congestive heart failure should supplement with magnesium. It is also beneficial in treating arrhythmia, including atrial fibrillation, PVC's and symptoms of mitral valve prolapse.

The Greatest Medicine

All of these natural approaches will benefit you greatly. But what will benefit you the most is your faith in God. He is a wonderful Creator of limitless power and imagination. Yet He loves you more deeply than you could ever imagine. Don't ever think your health does not matter to Him. Everything about you matters. The Bible says that He has even counted the number of hairs on your head! (See Luke 12:7.) He cares deeply about every infinite detail in your life—and His power is beyond your comprehension. Begin to speak His blessings and claim His healing.

> Praise the LORD, I tell myself; with my whole heart, I will praise his holy name. Praise the LORD, I tell myself, and never forget the good things he does for me. He forgives all my sins and heals all my diseases. He ransoms me from death and surrounds me with love and tender mercies. He fills my life with good things. My youth is renewed like the eagle's!
> —PSALM 103:1–5

We are pressed on every side by troubles, but we are not crushed and broken. We are perplexed, but we don't give up and quit. We are hunted down, but God never abandons us. We get knocked down, but we get up again and keep going. Through suffering, these bodies of ours constantly share in the death of Jesus so that the life of Jesus may also be seen in our bodies.

—2 Corinthians 4:8–10

Now, if you are trying the nutrients I've mentioned above and maintaining your close fellowship with the Lord, you might also think about another kind of therapy for treating your angina.

Have You Considered Chelation Therapy?

In 1956 Dr. Norman Clarke was treating a battery worker for lead poisoning using EDTA (ethylene diamine tetraacetic acid). After the patient had finished his treatment, the doctor noticed that the man's angina had also disappeared. Soon other doctors began following in Dr. Clarke's footsteps, and in 1972 the American College for the Advancement of Medicine was formed in order to educate physicians and to provide additional research for chelation therapy.[1]

Chelation therapy uses EDTA along with vitamins and minerals to improve blood flow and to purge the body of toxic heavy metals. Initially it was thought that EDTA unclogged arteries by removing the calcium out of the plaque. We now know that it improves blood flow by removing iron, copper, lead, cadmium and other toxic metals from the body. Doctors who administer chelation therapy recognize that arteriosclerosis not only affects the arteries of the heart, but also the smallest arteries and capillaries in the fingers, toes and throughout the entire body. In other words, the therapy improves blood flow throughout the entire body, whereas angioplasties and

> *I know how to live on almost nothing or with everything. I have learned the secret of living in every situation, whether it is with a full stomach or empty, with plenty or little. For I can do everything with the help of Christ who gives me the strength I need.*
> —PHILIPPIANS 4:12–13

coronary bypass grafts only treat small areas of arteriosclerosis.

Physicians have discovered that patients suffering from arteriosclerosis and lead poisoning reported surprising benefits from chelation. These benefits included: 1) patients were able to walk farther; 2) patients with angina were able to exercise more strenuously without developing chest pain; 3) patients with leg pain from poor circulation no longer experienced pain and were able to walk farther before leg pain developed. Along with these symptom-reducing benefits is the fact that EDTA also restores the normal production of prostacyclin, the prostaglandin hormone that prevents blood clots and arterial spasms, and improves blood flow, even in diseased arteries.

EDTA can also reduce the production of free radicals, which attack our cell structures and weaken our immune systems by as much as a million-fold! I believe that anyone with poor circulation, along with heavy metal toxicity (such as cadmium and lead) should consider having chelation therapy at least one time per week for twenty to forty treatments and then continue chelation therapy once a month as maintenance.[2]

Are You Looking Ahead?

One of the foundational problems involved with angina and other heart-disease conditions is poor circulation due to arteriosclerosis. It causes a diminished blood supply to vital organs of the body, including the brain, heart or kidneys. Poor blood supply, in turn, causes more plaque to form, which creates a vicious cycle and eventually leads to heart attack, stroke, kidney failure or possible amputation of an extremity.

To help, I recommend you follow the Balanced Carb-Protein-Fat Plan. Take a moment right now to flip to Appendix A in the back of this book and look over that plan. God knows the pain you feel from angina and has given you both spiritual and natural ways to end angina and walk in divine health. It's now up to you to step out in faith and apply the knowledge you have. As you jot down your Bible cure prescription, remember His healing promise: "I will give you back your health and heal your wounds, says the LORD" (Jer. 30:17).

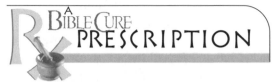

Marking Time With God

It's time to stop thinking about medicine for a little while! In a few minutes of silence, turn your thoughts to the Lord and meditate upon each verse below. When you're through, remain still and quiet before the Lord; consider your responses in His presence. How do they reveal the true desires of your heart? Your most pressing needs? Your greatest challenges as you confront heart disease? Simply underline the phrases that most apply to your situation and then pray asking God to meet your needs and heal your body.

Read each verse:

- Isaiah 41:10
- 1 Peter 5:10–11
- Philippians 3:20–21

If possible, during the coming week, share your Scripture markings with a family member, friend or pastor. Talk about them together, and then encourage one another.

Chapter 5

Hope to Overcome Hypertension

Y ou may have just discovered that you have high blood pressure *(hypertension)*, or you may already be taking medication for it. Hypertension is often called the silent killer since it often goes for years without being detected.

I have good news for you. God has created a number of natural ways to lower or keep your high blood pressure within normal limits. We will explore these together. Be certain to consult with your doctor before taking any new steps. And be certain to consult with God for His healing power and guidance in your life.

A BIBLE CURE PRAYER
FOR YOU

Almighty God, heal my body and lower my blood pressure. I speak to my heart and entire circulatory system to be healed in Jesus' name. Lord, I ask for Your guidance in the right steps to take to lower my blood pressure and to live by faith, not doubt; by hope, not discouragement; and to live in divine health, not sickness, in Jesus' name. Amen.

Checking Out Your Pressure

You absolutely need to know whether you have high blood pressure. Left untreated, it can wreak the kind of destruction on your heart and arteries that, over the years, can make you a major risk for both heart attacks and strokes.

Studies estimate that one out of four adults in the United States is battling high blood pressure, and more than 30 percent are completely unaware of their condition. Many of these folks display no symptoms at all and often go undiagnosed and untreated for years.

Regular blood pressure screening can help you receive an early diagnosis and treatment, which greatly reduces the risks of further complications.

Now, do you have high blood pressure? I recommend seeing your doctor to find out. But you can probably get a ballpark figure on your blood pressure with the machine at your local drugstore. Here's how high blood pressure, or hypertension, is defined by the numbers.

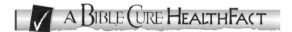

Categories for Blood Pressure Levels in Adults

- *Borderline hypertension* is defined as systolic blood pressure between 120 and 160, and diastolic blood pressure between 90 and 94.
- *Mild hypertension* is defined as systolic blood pressure between 140 and 160, and diastolic between 95 and 104.
- *Moderate hypertension* is defined as systolic blood pressure between 140 and 180, and diastolic blood pressure between 105 and 114.
- *Severe hypertension* is defined as systolic blood pressure greater than 160, and diastolic greater than 115.

Generally speaking, having a systolic reading greater than 140 and diastolic reading greater than 90 means you should look into the matter further. Many cases of high blood pressure can be completely controlled through diet and lifestyle changes. However, patients with severe hypertension should be on antihypertensive medication such as an ACE inhibitor. The Joint National Committee on Detection, Evaluation and Treatment of High Blood Pressure recommends that non-drug therapies be used to treat borderline to mild hypertension. About half of the people with high blood pressure fall into this category.[1]

If you do discover that you have high blood pressure, don't be discouraged. You can easily find out how serious your condition is, and then learn what to do about it.

Lowering and Controlling Blood Pressure

Why lower and/or control your blood pressure? For one thing, controlling high blood pressure can prevent congestive heart failure. This form of heart disease is usually due to a weakness in the heart muscle, making it unable to pump effectively. The cause may be a previous heart attack, long-term hypertension or a cardiomyopathy (a disease of the heart muscle).

Symptoms include extreme weakness, fatigue and shortness of breath, especially after mild to moderate exercise. Congestive heart failure is quite common in the elderly population and is often treated with Lasix, a strong diuretic. Use of Lasix, however, can cause a thiamine deficiency. If you are a patient with congestive heart failure on Lasix, take generous amounts of B-complex vitamins, especially thiamine, in a dose of at least 200 milligrams a day. Individuals with congestive heart failure may need to limit their fluids, too. (It's important to remain under the care of a cardiologist and a good nutritional doctor as you battle this condition.)

As with most conditions involving the health of

> *Don't worry about anything; instead, pray about everything. Tell God what you need, and thank him for all he has done. If you do this, you will experience God's peace, which is far more wonderful than the human mind can understand. His peace will guard your hearts and minds as you live in Christ Jesus.*
> —PHILIPPIANS 4:6–7

your cardiovascular system, certain lifestyle choices play a significant role in prevention or control of hypertension. These include cutting out smoking and alcohol drinking, limiting stress, taking up exercise and cutting down on the caffeine. Eating habits that contribute to hypertension include eating too much salt, sugar and saturated fats, while not eating enough fiber and not taking in enough potassium, magnesium and calcium.

You can make lifestyle changes to lower your blood pressure through Christ's help. You are not alone in this. He will both encourage and empower you by His Spirit not only to make healthy decisions about how you live and what you eat but also to follow through on your decision. Take time to say this verse out loud often today and claim His strength in your new lifestyle: "For I can do everything with the help of Christ who gives me the strength I need" (Phil. 4:13).

Specifically, please do at least the following four things to keep hypertension at bay.

1. Maintain Your Ideal Weight

Maintaining your ideal body weight is one of the most important factors in lowering blood pressure. If you need to lose weight, I recommend the Balanced Carb-Protein-Fat Plan listed at the end of this book.

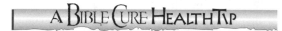

A BIBLE CURE HEALTH TIP

Keys for Weight Loss

- Drink two quarts of filtered or bottled water a day. It is best to drink two 8-oz. glasses thirty minutes before each meal, or one to two 8-oz. glasses 2½ hours after each meal.
- Consult your doctor about getting on a regular exercise program.
- Avoid sugar.
- You may eat fruit, however, avoid fruit juices.
- Avoid alcohol.
- Avoid all fried foods.
- Avoid, or decrease dramatically, starches. Starches include all breads, crackers, bagels, potatoes, pasta, rice, corn and black, pinto and red beans. Also limit intake of bananas.
- Eat fresh fruits; steamed, stir-fried or raw vegetables; lean meats; salads, preferably with extra-virgin olive oil and vinegar; nuts (almonds, organic peanuts) and seeds.
- Fiber supplements such as Fiber Plus, Perdiem Fiber or any other fiber without NutraSweet or sugar.

- Take 2 tablespoons of milk of magnesia each day if constipated.
- For snacks, choose Iron Man PR Bars, Zone Bars or Balance Bars. My favorite snack bar is the yogurt honey peanut balance bars. These may be purchased at a health food store.
- Do not eat past 7 P.M.
- Check with your physician or nutritional doctor before implementing any new plan.

2. Transform Your Diet

There will be some things to cut out and some things to add. Begin by eating more fruits and vegetables. Plant foods have much higher amounts of potassium and lower amounts of sodium. They also provide essential fatty acids, fiber, calcium, magnesium and vitamin C. Eating fresh, natural foods, including lots of fruits and vegetables, brings powerful benefits to the hypertensive person.

And why not start using a juicer? You can juice carrots, apples, parsley and celery, once or twice a day. Drink at least a half a cup a day of organic celery juice, since it has been discovered that celery can lower blood pressure.

Other foods that may help lower blood pressure include:

- onions and garlic

- green leafy vegetables

- salmon

- mackerel and other cold-water fish

- high-fiber foods such as whole grains and legumes

Here are a few more important health steps you can take to lower your blood pressure:

Increase your potassium intake, and decrease your salt intake, because a diet high in sodium and low in potassium is associated with hypertension. Most potassium is found inside the body's cells, whereas the majority of sodium is found outside of the body's cells. Processed foods contain high amounts of sodium, and even more

> *For God has not given us a spirit of fear and timidity, but of power, love, and self-discipline.*
> —2 TIMOTHY 1:7

sodium is added during the cooking process.

Americans add only a small amount of sodium to their food from the salt shaker, so most of it comes from the processed foods we buy and the salt that we add during cooking. Reduce your consumption of processed foods and salt. It's because of these processed foods that most Americans take in twice as much sodium as potassium. We should be taking in

> So I tell you, don't worry about everyday life whether you have enough food, drink, and clothes. Doesn't life consist of more than food and clothing? Look at the birds. They don't need to plant or harvest or put food in barns because your heavenly Father feeds them. And you are far more valuable to him than they are.
> —MATTHEW 6:25–26

five times as much potassium as sodium. The only way to insure this balance is to juice fruits and vegetables regularly or to increase our intake of fruits and vegetables.[2]

You may also take potassium supplements while decreasing your intake of processed foods. A good way to get your potassium is to use the brand *NoSalt* (or any other similar variety of salt substitute) that contains 530 milligrams of potassium per one-sixth teaspoon. You can take one and a half to three grams of potassium salts a day. A dose of 400 milligrams of magnesium three times a day may also lower blood pressure. Always consult your physician before taking either magnesium or potassium.

Vitamin C may also lower blood pressure by helping the body to eliminate heavy metals such as lead. The recommended daily allowance for adults is 60 milligrams, however, I recommend 100 to 300 milligrams a day.

Garlic may also lower blood pressure. I recommend taking a dose of 400 milligrams of garlic, three times a day, or 4,000 micrograms of allicin content three times a day.

Vitamin B_6 may also be helpful in lowering blood pressure. This may be due to its diuretic effects, or by the reduction of norepinephrine levels. The dose of B_6 is 50 to 100 milligrams per day.

Fish oil and flaxseed oil is also effective in keeping blood pressure levels low. One tablespoon of flaxseed oil, once or twice a day, or three capsules of fish oil three times a day, are both very effective in lowering blood pressure.

Coenzyme Q₁₀ may also reduce blood pressure in a dose of 100 to 200 milligrams a day.

Asparagus tablets help to reduce blood pressure. Asparagus is a natural diuretic and is taken in a dose of two tablets, three times a day.

Chelation therapy can also lower blood pressure by binding heavy metals, such as lead and cadmium, so the body can excrete them through the kidneys. I have witnessed peoples' blood pressures decreasing dramatically after they've undergone chelation therapy treatments.

These dietary changes and lifestyle changes can dramatically impact your blood pressure. After consulting your doctor, try a combination of these recommendations and discover new hope for beating high blood pressure.

3. Get Involved in Regular Exercise

When was the last time you got out of the house and walked, jogged or bicycled around the block? Or are you participating in any type of regular, moderate form of exertion? It's time to get up out of that chair and get active! Regular exercise is one of the best ways to maintain good health. Exercise pumps oxygen to your cells, giving your body added ability to win the war against heart disease. Of course, any exercise program should be under the supervision of your doctor.

4. Decrease Stress

One natural step for reducing stress is taking 70 milligrams of kava three times a day, or 5-HTP (hydroxy-L-tryptophan), 50 to 100 milligrams, three times a day with meals. 5-HTP should not be taken with other antidepressants such as Prozac, Zoloft or Paxil.

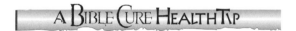

A BIBLE CURE HEALTH TIP

Decrease Stress

Decrease stress by meditating on the Word of God, especially scriptures about peace like this one: "Let the Holy Spirit fill and control you. Then you will sing psalms and hymns and spiritual songs among yourselves, making music to the Lord in your hearts. And you will always give thanks for everything to God the Father in the name of our Lord Jesus Christ" (Eph. 5:19–20).

Also, you can reduce stress by living more for others. Taking up a less me-centered existence means less worry and a less controlling approach toward life's events. Paul lived a life crucified to self: "I myself no longer live, but Christ lives in me. So I live my life in this earthly body by trusting in the Son of God, who loved me and gave himself for me" (Gal. 2:20). Ask yourself today, "How can I love others and live for Christ and not myself?" Take the focus off yourself and your problems and fix your eyes on Christ (Heb. 12:1–2).

Offering a Little Encouragement

We've now come to the end of this little booklet on heart disease. I hope you've found some hope and encouragement in these pages. I know that having heart disease of any kind can be a fearful thing, but the scriptural and medical principles in this booklet really can make a difference. I want to encourage you, though, to look to God for the strength and wisdom to begin taking a few first steps toward change. Even if your cardiovascular system is relatively healthy at this point, making some of the nutritional changes

I've recommended can make all the difference to your future.

But whatever your situation, please remember that your life, with all its joys and sorrows, is always held close to God's own heart. Your heart matters to His! So trust in His goodness for today, tomorrow and each day thereafter. He cares for you, and His promise is never to leave you. (See Matthew 28:20.) That is the greatest promise you could ever have.

Trust in the Lord

> Let the smile of your face shine on us, LORD. You have given me greater joy than those who have abundant harvests of grain and wine. I will lie down in peace and sleep, for you alone, O Lord, will keep me safe.
>
> —PSALM 4:5–8

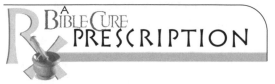

Recap Your Progress

In light of all you've learned, list three things you are NOT doing now that you need to do to lower the risk of heart disease in your future:

1. _____
2. _____
3. _____

List 3 things you ARE doing right that you need to keep doing:

1. _____
2. _____
3. _____

Jot down three Scripture passages that build hope in you as you overcome heart disease:

_____

_____

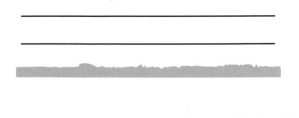

The Balanced Carb-Protein-Fat Plan

There is no perfect diet for everyone. A regimen that's healthy for one individual may actually be harmful to another due to food allergies, food sensitivities, gastrointestinal disturbances, blood types and other factors.

The diet of the majority of people in the United States contains excessive amounts of fat, sugar, salt and starch, and it has a significant lack of fiber. The keys to the ultimate healthy lifestyle are found in eating primarily fruits, vegetables, whole grains, nuts, seeds, beans, legumes and lean meats.

Avoid refined sugar and flour; avoid fats, which include hydrogenated fats, saturated fats and heat processed polyunsaturated fats such as luncheon meats, cured meats and sausage; and avoid foods high in salt. Also, limit your intake of red meat, choosing the leanest cuts possible.

The nutritional plan I recommend to my patients is the Balanced Carb-Protein-Fat Plan. Here's how it works. Each time you eat you should combine foods in a ratio of 40 percent carbohydrates, 30 percent proteins and 30 percent fats.

This program balances the correct ratio of carbohydrates, proteins and fats, thereby controlling insulin.

Elevated insulin levels decrease physical performance and are one of the primary predictors used in evaluating a person's risk of developing heart disease. To simplify this program, I will list the food categories and blocks, and then demonstrate how to use the blocks through the day. Let's look at some comparisons.

- One block of protein is equal to 7 grams of protein, which is equivalent to approximately 1 oz. of meat, such as beef, chicken breast, turkey breast and so on.

- One block of carbohydrates is equal to 9 grams of carbohydrates, which is equivalent to ½ slice of bread, ¼ bagel, ⅕ cup of rice, ⅓ banana, ½ apple or ¼ cup of pasta. This will be explained in greater detail later.

- One block of fat is equal to 1½ grams of fat, which is equivalent to ⅓ tsp. of olive oil, 6 peanuts, 3 almonds, 1 tbsp. of avocado and so on.

You will be getting much larger portion sizes than each individual food block. In fact, the average sedentary woman will get three food blocks at each meal plus one food block midmorning, one food block midafternoon and one food block at bedtime. An active female who exercises three to four times a week for at least thirty minutes, may have four food blocks with each meal and one food block between meals and at bedtime.

A sedentary male may have four food blocks at each meal and one food block between meals and at bedtime, whereas the active male, who exercises three to four times a week, may have five to six food blocks at each meal and one food block between meals and at bedtime.

Let's discuss the different food blocks—starting with protein.

Protein Blocks

(Approximately 7 grams of protein for each block)

Meats

One ounce of skinless chicken breast, skinless turkey breast or free range chicken. Or 1 ounce of skinless dark meat of turkey, skinless dark meat of chicken, hamburger with less than 10 percent fat, lean pork chop, lean ham, lean Canadian bacon, lean lamb or veal. Note: I do not recommend eating pork and ham regularly. If an individual has a degenerative disease, he or she should avoid these meats completely.

Fish

Eat 1½ oz. of the following:

Salmon	Mackerel
Orange roughy	Red snapper
Sole	Mahi-mahi
Trout	Halibut
Grouper	

Eggs, dairy products and soy protein

Eggs—one whole egg or three egg whites
Dairy products—1 oz. low fat cheese, ¼ cup of low-fat cottage cheese
Soy protein—⅓ oz. of protein powder, ¼ soy burger, 3 oz. of tofu

Carbohydrate Blocks

(Approximately 9 grams of carbohydrates for each block)

Fruit

1 tangerine, lemon, lime, kiwi or peach
½ apple, orange, grapefruit, pear or nectarine
⅓ banana
1 cup strawberries, raspberries
⅓ cup cubed watermelon, cubed cantaloupe
½ cup cubed honeydew melon, cherries, black-
berries, blueberries, grapes, cubed pineapples,
papaya
⅓ cup applesauce, mango

Juice

¼ cup grape, pineapple
⅓ cup apple, grapefruit, orange, lemon
¾ cup V8

Cooked Vegetables

⅛ cup baked beans
⅕ cup sweet potatoes or mashed potatoes
¼ cup lentils, kidney beans, black beans, red
beans, lima beans, pinto beans, refried beans,
corn
⅓ cup peas, baked potato
1 cup asparagus, green beans, carrots
1¼ cup broccoli, spinach, squash
1⅓ cup cabbage

Cooked Vegetables

1½ cup zucchini, Brussels sprouts, eggplant
1¾ cup turnip greens
2 cups cauliflower, collard greens

Raw Vegetables

1 cucumber
2 tomatoes
1 cup onions (chopped), snow peas
1½ cup broccoli
2 cups cauliflower
2½ cups celery, green peppers (chopped)
3 cups cabbage, mushrooms (chopped)
4 cups romaine lettuce (chopped), cucumber (sliced)
6 cups spinach

Grains

⅕ oz. brown or white rice
⅕ cup cooked pasta
⅓ cup cooked oatmeal (or ½ oz. dry), or grits
¼ bagel, English muffin
½ biscuit, waffle, or ½ of a 4-inch pancake, flour tortilla
½ oz. dry cereal
1 rice cake or corn tortilla
4 saltine crackers

High-Sugar Items

½ tbsp. honey or molasses
2 tsp. maple syrup
2 tbsp. ketchup, jelly (choose fructose jelly)

Fat Blocks

⅓ tsp. almond butter, olive oil, canola oil, flax-seed oil

⅓ tsp. natural peanut butter

1 tsp. olive oil and vinegar dressing, light mayonnaise, chopped walnuts

1 tbsp. avocado, guacamole

1 whole macadamia nut

1½ tsp. almond (slivered)

3 almonds, olives, pistachios, cashews

6 peanuts

The Basics

An example of a meal with four food blocks would be 4 oz. of chicken (equal to four protein blocks); 1 cup of cooked asparagus, 1 head of lettuce and 1 cup of red beans (all together equal to four carbohydrates blocks); 1 tablespoon of olive oil and vinegar dressing (equal to four fat blocks).

To simplify this meal plan even more, picture the palm of your hand and imagine placing a piece of protein (such as a piece of chicken, turkey, fish or lean red meat) the size of your palm. Next cup your hands and picture putting in the amount of vegetables or fruit that you can hold. You should add 12 almonds, 12 cashews or 12 pistachio nuts or 24 peanuts. You are holding the ingredients for your healthy meal.

It's best to dramatically limit starches, which include bread, bagels, crackers, pasta, rice, pretzels, popcorn, beans, cereals, corn, potatoes, potato chips, corn chips and any other starchy item. I recommend grazing through the day, eating a fairly large breakfast, lunch and dinner and smaller midmorning, midafternoon and evening snacks. Eat the evening meal before 7 P.M.

People who have degenerative diseases such as heart disease, high blood pressure, high cholesterol, diabetes, hypoglycemia, cancer or patients who desire optimal health should closely follow the Balanced Carb-Protein-Fat Plan program.

If the Balanced Carb-Protein-Fat Plan program seems too complicated for you, simply follow these basic instructions:

1.   Reduce the intake of high starch foods, including bread, crackers, bagels, pretzels, corn, popcorn, potatoes,

sweet potatoes, potato chips, pasta, rice, beans and bananas. Better yet, eliminate them all together.

2. Avoid all simple sugar food such as candies, cookies, cakes, pies and donuts. If you must have sugar use Sweet Balance or Stevia, a sweetener made from kiwi fruit. Choose fruit instead of fruit juices.

3. Increase your intake of nonstarchy vegetables such as spinach, lettuce, cabbage, broccoli, asparagus, green beans and cauliflower.

4. Choose healthy proteins such as turkey breast, chicken breast, fish, free-range beef, low-fat cottage cheese and so on. Select healthy fats such as nuts, seeds, flaxseed oil, extra-virgin olive oil or small amounts of organic butter. Use extra-virgin olive oil and vinegar as a salad dressing. Choose the healthy fats we have listed instead of polyunsaturated, saturated and hydrogenated fats.

5. Eat three meals a day consisting of fruit, nonstarchy vegetables, lean meat and good fat. You should also have a healthy midmorning, midafternoon and evening snack.

By following these guidelines I believe you will experience increased energy and improved health.

Appendix B

Chelation Therapy

There are diverse opinions about chelation therapy. Here is the official statement of the American Heart Association concerning chelation therapy as posted at their Web site at www.americanheart.org in 1999.

> The American Heart Association has reviewed the available literature on the use of chelation (E.D.T.A., ethylenediamine tetraacetic acid) in treating arteriosclerotic heart disease. They found no scientific evidence to demonstrate any benefit from this form of therapy.
>
> Chelation therapy is a recognized treatment for heavy metal (such as lead)

poisoning. E.D.T.A., injected into the blood, will bind the metals and allow them to be removed from the body in the urine. There have been no adequate, controlled, published scientific studies using currently approved scientific methodology to support this therapy. The United States Food and Drug Administration (FDA), the National Institutes of Health (NIH) and the American College of Cardiology all agree with the AHA on this point. Furthermore, using this form of unproven treatment may deprive patients of the well-established benefits from the many other valuable methods of treating these diseases.

A recent study of chelation therapy, using currently approved scientific methodology, determined that EDTA chelation therapy was no more effective than a placebo (sugar pill) in treating men and women with peripheral vascular disease of the legs (intermittent claudication).

Thus, there still is no scientific evidence that demonstrates any benefit from this form of therapy.

There are, however, multitudes of individual testimonies that support this therapy. If you are considering chelation therapy, I would encourage you to do your own research on chelation therapy and draw your own conclusion as to what would be best for you. If you have heavy metal toxicity, such as excessive amounts of lead, cadmium, etc. on a six- hour urine test after taking a chelation agent such as DMSA or EDTA, then you would probably benefit from chelation therapy. If you had heavy metal toxicity along with peripheral vascular disease or coronary artery disease, then it is possible that the peripheral vascular disease and the coronary artery disease may be improved with the chelation of heavy metals.

Notes

PREFACE
THERE'S HOPE FOR YOUR HEART

1. Statistics from the American Heart Association Web site at www.americanheart.com.

CHAPTER 1
HOPE TO BEAT THE STATISTICS FOR HEART DISEASE

1. Statistics from the American Heart Association Web site at www.americanheart.com.

CHAPTER 2
HOPE TO OVERCOME THE RISK OF HEART DISEASE

1. "Diagonal Earlobe Creases and Prognosis of Patients With Suspected Coronary Artery Disease," American Medical Journal, Med 100 (1996): 205–211.
2. M. Friedman, *Treating Type A Behavior and Your Heart* (n.p., Ballantine Books, 1984), 33–43.
3. S. I. McMillen, *None of These Diseases* (Westwood, NJ: Revell, 1963), 115.

CHAPTER 3
HOPE FOR LOWER CHOLESTEROL

1. James F. Balch, M.D., and Phyllis A. Balch, C.N.C., *Prescription for Nutritional Healing,* (Garden City, NY: Avery Publishing Group, 1997).
2. Friedensohn, Aharon, et al., "Malignant Arrhythmias in Relation to Values of Serum Potassium in Patients With Acute Myocardial Infarction," *International Journal of Cardiology 32,* (1991) 331–338.
3. You can read more about this therapy in Dr.

Nambudripad's book, *Say Goodbye to Illness,* available on the Internet at www.naet.com.

4. M. J. Stampfer et al., "Vitamin E Consumption and the Risk of Coronary Disease in Women," *New England Journal of Medicine 328* (1993): 1444–1448.

5. E. B. Rimm, "Vitamin E Consumption and the Risk of Coronary Heart Disease in Men," *New England Journal of Medicine 328* (1993): 1430.

CHAPTER 4
HOPE FOR ENDING ANGINA

1. N. E. Clarke et al., "Treatment of Angina Pectoris with Dissodium Ethylene Diamine Tetraacetic Acid," *American Medical Journal of Medical Science 232* (1956): 654.

2. Please note that there is some controversy surrounding the use of chelation therapy. For example, it is FDA approved for lead poisoning but not for arteriosclerosis. Carefully read my note in Appendix B. And if you'd like to look into this therapy further, I recommend the following book: Elmer Cranton, M.D., *Bypassing Bypass* (Troutdale, VA: Medex Publishers, 1990).

CHAPTER 5
HOPE TO OVERCOME HYPERTENSION

1. The Sixth Report of the Joint National Committee on Prevention, Detection, Evaluation and Treatment of High Blood Pressure authored by the National Heart, Lung and Blood Institutes of Health, published in *NIH Publication No. 98* 4080, (Nov. 1997).

2. H.G. Langford, "Dietary Potassium and Hypertension: Epidemiological Data," *Ann Intern Med 98* (1990): 770–2.

Don Colbert, M.D., was born in Tupelo, Mississippi. He attended Oral Roberts School of Medicine in Tulsa, Oklahoma, where he received a bachelor of science degree in biology in addition to his degree in medicine. Dr. Colbert completed his internship and residency with Florida Hospital in Orlando, Florida. He is board certified in family practice and has received extensive training in nutritional medicine.

If you would like more
information about natural and
divine healing, or information about
Divine Health Nutritional Products®,
you may contact
Dr. Colbert at:

DR. DON COLBERT

1908 Boothe Circle
Longwood, FL 32750
Telephone: 407-331-7007

Dr. Colbert's website is
www.drcolbert.com.

BIBLE CURE

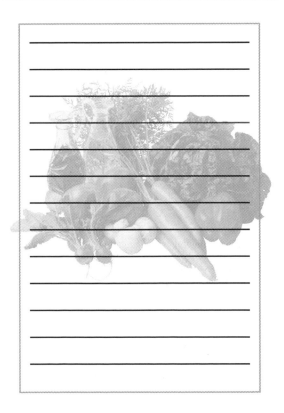

_____

_____

_____

_____

_____

_____

_____

_____

_____

_____

_____

_____